1. Natural beauty on your face

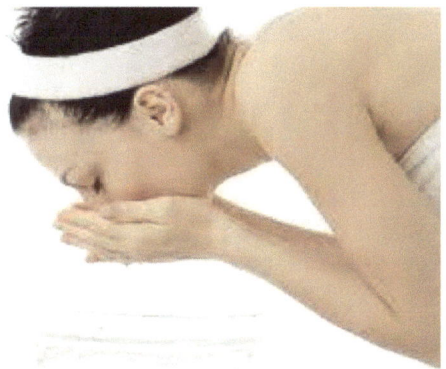

The following are the natural facial wash technique:

1. Apply water gently on your face.
2. Apply the gentle daily cleansing gel on the hand then put on the forehead inside out & from right to left for left side of the forehead & left to right for right side of the forehead.
3. Use your whole palm to hold your face from inside out with your smiling face from inside out & from right to left for left side of the face & left to right for right side of the face
4. Clean your nose area from top to bottom.
5. Clean your upper lips from inside out & from right to left for left side of the upper lips & left to right for right side of the upper lips.
6. Do the same for your chin.
7. Clean your neck from bottom to top & from left to right & right to left.
8. Splashing water on your face & use water to clean your neck from bottom to top & from left to right & right to left.
9. Use the Scrub by following the technique same as the 2 to 7 steps.
10. Splash water on your face & use water to clean your neck from bottom to top & from left to right & right to left. Use sponge to absorb the water from your face.
11. Spray the Misting Gel.
12. Apply the Serum on your face using the same technique as 2 to 7 steps.
13. Apply the Moisturizing on your face using the same technique as 2 to 7 steps.
14. Apply the eye gel by circle clock wise with finger & massage the eye inside out & from right to left for left side of the eye & left to right for right side of the eye.

Hope you enjoy this unique Facial care technique for every morning & night.

2. Weight Management

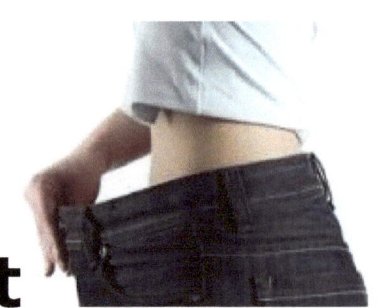

My dear friends, how many of you wanted to have an ideal weight?

I am sure everyone wanted to have ideal weight, right?

However, most of us when we expose to favorites foods we will forget about

our ideal weight mission, right?

It is normal.

Hence, we need to answer the following question:

1.Why you need an ideal weight?

2.Seek someone to remind you if you are tempted to eat more than you need.

3.Ask yourselves whether you eat to live or live to eat?

4.What happen if your body system breakdown because you eat too much to create burden to your body system?

5.Put the ideal weight picture in your wallet & in front of the mirror(compare now with the ideal picture) to remind yourselves on the mission to achieve the ideal weight.

6.Formula for weight management = Prefer white meat+ vegetables+ daily exercise for 20 minutes (walking/running/climb stairs/jumping)

8.Dinner eat vegetables or fruits before 8pm.

9.Imagine you have achieved the ideal weight what would you get. Please write it down & keep it in your wallet where you can see every time you open your wallet.

The above are combination formula or recipe from friends who successfully loose weight with combination of my recipe.

3. External & internal maintenance

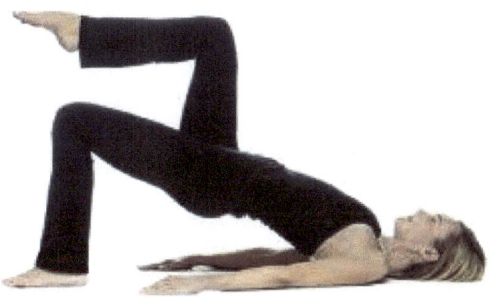

Well as we all know, our body system need variety of the vitamins in the body from top to bottom correct? That is call internal maintenance only.

Similarly, for our external maintenance means skin care & facial care.

Let me ask you how often you service your car?

Why you need engine oil & service car?

Similarly, your body system, skin & face need maintenance too. Imagine what happen if you are not maintaining your car engine & not send car for service?

What happen if the car engine is damaged?

For car we may replace the engine or repair the engine.

However if our body organ is damaged or system is damaged can we replace or repair it ?

How our family choose our product & what we eat since young.

I wish to send a **BIG THANK YOU to my PARENTS** because of them I got this secret from young and I done a lot of reading to top up the knowledge too.

How many people know how to select the good product for themselves?

Your results of internal body system & external results will tell you the answer.

Results mean your **face & skin & your medical record**.

Why I could share with you, mainly I already got the results of **18 years old** body system & my face & skin is around that age too? My actual age is almost 38 **years old.**

My intention here is to create Awareness of how to maintain Natural Young **to you from inside out.**

Is it possible when you are 60 or 70 years old you are as energetic as 18 years old boys or girl?

My Answer is definitely YES.

Tell you about my father already 60 plus my mum is around the age too. They are still as energetic as the youngster.

When I look at their energy level, it is possible to be energetic at that age too.

How many of you want that?

Do you want that so that you can do whatever you like when you were young without hire or depend on others to take care you which cost money either in medical cost or hire someone to look after you which can be trusted.

Imagine you are at age 60 or 70 you still can travel everywhere with your young look & body system?

Is it amazing?

Actually, I felt really bad when I saw my similar age friends or relatives look older and I wish to share this secret to more people so that they could get the same result that I get before it is too late.

Today I myself am the **Evidence** to all of you at any age we could still look & have the body system of 18years old.

It is only one thing whether you give the reason on not to do it or you want the results then you choose to do that.

Stay tune with me.

4. Sweats to Beauty

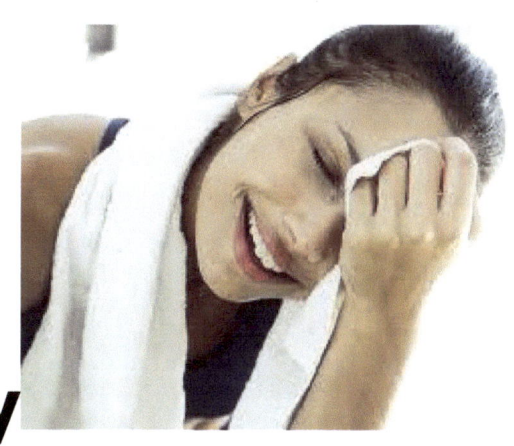

Hahaha do you like natural perfume?

Let me share with you my natural perfume..

What??wait wait wait...answer a few question before you run away...:)

How often do you sweat?

How many type of activities could create sweat?

1. Sport/exercise
2. Drink soup
3. Steam bath or saunas in the spa
4. Eat hot food
5. Hot weather

Do you know, actually sweat is good to purify your skin & getting toxic out of your skin.

It promotes good health because remove toxic, beauty & weight loss, improve mood by making us more relax, improve cardiovascular health.

Sweating could get rid of harmful substances like alcohol, cholesterol and salt.

Well, let's enjoy the natural perfume together.

Before we sweats if we drink the GRN then it helps to remove the toxic from the inside out.

Hope you enjoy sweats in future.

See you in next recipe!

5. Clear skin on face & body

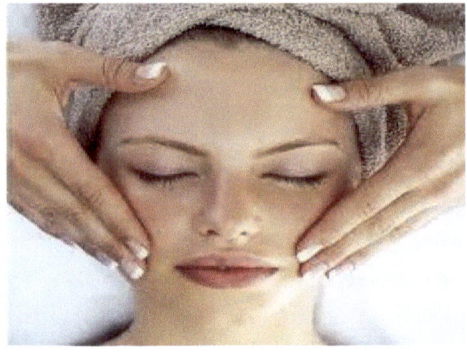

Whew...looking forward to see you here, luckily today i can make it's a professional accountant in MNC company, i am involving in many other activities to improve myself both skin, body & mind & skills.

Therefore, it is time consuming for me to write such a long articles to share with you.

However, i miss you & wanted to help more people to achieve the results that i have achieved so i am committed to this..

Hahaha.. you must have missing me already, right?

Have you seen girls who can meet you with the TRUE face on day & night?

Well girls or guys, you start wondering those who is with cosmetic what is their TRUE FACE right?Eeeee.. me tooo...

I heard a story from my friend who told me one jokes, a man who got married to a girl who used to be with cosmetic, and he could not recognized her without the cosmetic.

It is fine to be with cosmetic, however, how to maintain young skin & face even after using colourful cosmetic.

Well, there is a magic here!!

I am sharing with you on the secret of having a clear skin on face & body.

It sounds interesting & exciting to share with you my fellows friends!

Formula are as follows:

1. EAT FORMULA: **TOMATOES +APPLES + WATER**
2. SKIN CARE FORMULA: **SUNBLOCK SPF 30 + AVOID HOT SUN + SWEATS FROM FACE & BODY + SKIN CARE PRODUCTS + CLEAN FACE PROPERLY AFTER COSMETIC**

My dear friends, the above formula can help people to clear the pigmentation on the skin.

6. Breathing

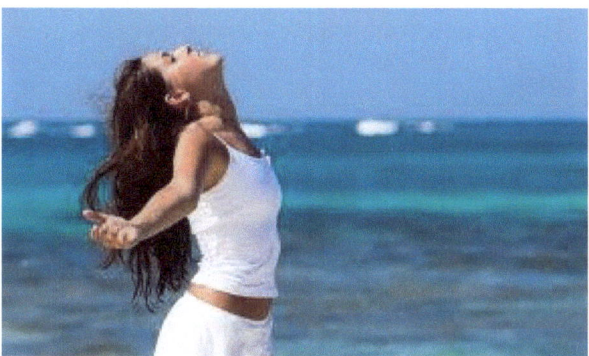

Thank you so much to all my friends here who give lots of supports.

Therefore, today i am sharing my technique of exercise & relax anytime anywhere to show my appreciation to all of you.

You are wondering what kind of exercise can be done in anytime & anywhere correct.

Actually, if we breathing in slowly & deeply it will helps us to keep our stomach in & it exercise our chest & stomach together.

Then, we breathe out and release it with an "ahhhhhhh" sound with maximum release level in a relaxing manner & feel the comfort of doing that. Immediately, we felt better.

I advise you, you may do this early in the morning with fresh air as it gives our body with fresh air which is very important to supply oxygen and as an energy production process which is called metabolism. You may put on some soothing music to do this stomach & chest exercise.

If we continuously to do this, we will get enough oxygen which generate healthy cells and will bring us healthy body.

Hope you benefits from this breathing exercise & see you in next recipe.

7. Beauty Masks

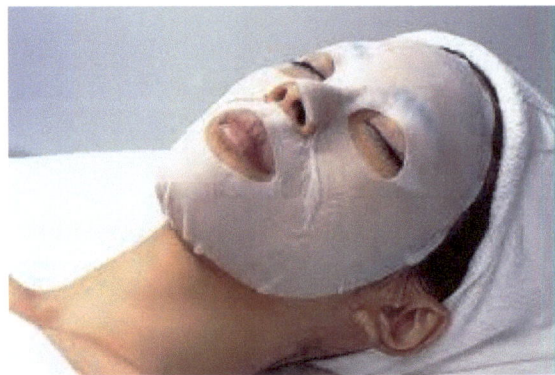

People use to ask me how i maintain my face..

Actually, it is all about i know how to choose the facial product and i change my facial product quite frequently.

I have chosen product on my face with masks to maintain my facial beside my daily skin care product. I understand that my face and skin needs multivitamin too.

Hope you get this tips.

Feel free to join us at facebook on:

1. http://www.facebook.com/#!/YoungRecipe

2. http://www.facebook.com/naturalbeautyrecipe?ref=hl

8. How you clean your internal organ?

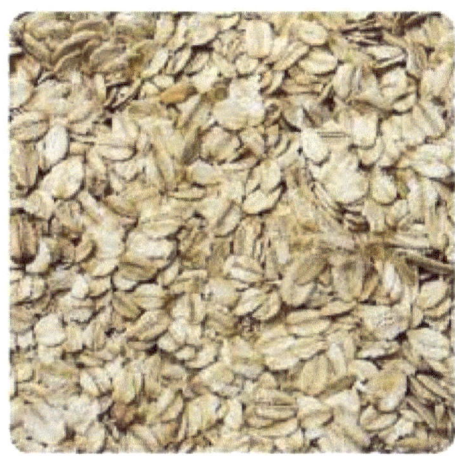

How to have forever young internal organ?

Have you heard of Oat?

I think everyone heard about it, actually oat help us to clean the cholesterol in our body.

The oats help to clean body toxic & chemical that we consume daily.

Besides all the daily food that we consume OAT help to maintain our body organ.

9. Maintain Healthy liver daily

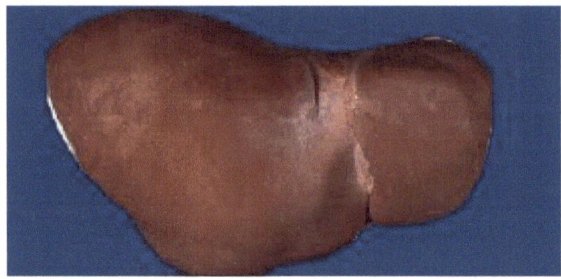

As age grow we use to worry about how to maintain our youth both internal organ and external beauty.

Here is some tips on maintain healthy liver daily:

1. Garlic and anion

Garlic helps the liver rid the body of mercury, certain food additives and the hormone oestrogen.

2. vegetables (broccoli, Brussel sprouts, cauliflower, cabbage).

These vegetables are very powerful detoxifiers of the liver.

3. Apples

This reduces the load on the liver and its detoxification capacities.

4. Bitter leafy salad greens

The bitterness of these foods helps to stimulate bile flow within the liver.

5. Soyabean

It can prevent and/or reduce the risk of a multitude of things like: breast cancer, heart disease, stroke and osteoporosis.

6. Oats

The health benefits of oats reach far beyond just cholesterol controlling; eating oats on a regular basis may reduce heart disease risk, prevent type 2 diabetes, and reduce carcinogens in the gastrointestinal tract.

7.Goji Berries

It is soothing yet powerful health promoting tonic.

Hope it helps.

10. Natural beauty skin

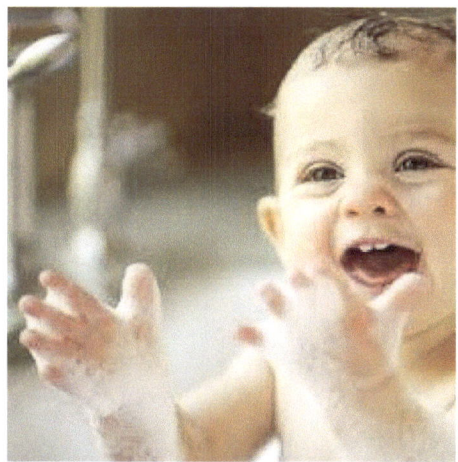

Best Vegetables to Better and Beautify Your Skin

1. Spinach.

The green leafs provide more nutrients on average than most other foods. Skin helping nutrients include Vitamin E, Vitamin A, and many B vitamins.

2. Sweet Potatoes.

Switch out your baked potato for a side of the sweet. A single sweet potato contains over 200% of your daily Vitamin A needs.

3. Turnip Greens.

Green turnip contains high levels of Vitamins K, A, and E, while keeping a low calorie count.

4. Carrots.

Not only good for the eyes, but the Vitamin A in carrots can help your skin. They also contain a large amount of Vitamin C and fiber.

5. Tomato

It contains antioxidants, in addition to vitamins A and C.

6. Papaya

Papaya is a natural exfoliating tonic. It leaves your skin spotless with its high vitamin A content.

11. Neck Care

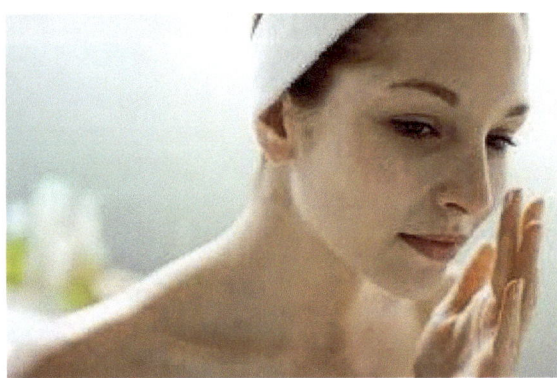

You wonder why Giraffe neck is here right?

You are looking forward to see me here & stretch the neck until like Giraffe's neck already...

Let me share some tips to massage your giraffe neck later ok!

Now i am sharing a jokes with you, when i was in college, one of my friend A ask friend B the following questions.

A: You have curry chicken yesterday, right?

B: How you know?

Me: Me too i have curry chicken yesterday.

A & B look at my neck. I wonder why they look at my neck..Hahaha

B: You do not eat curry chicken!

Me: Who said, I have curry chicken yesterday afternoon.

A & B laugh nonstop..

Me: Why both of you laugh? The curry chicken was delicious.

A &B & C & etc laugh nonstop..

My dear friends, do you know why they laugh & what they mean?

Guess why they laugh & what they mean!

Yes, they referred to "love bite" while else i referred to "curry chicken".

Do you know neck care is very important?

Actually, we need to take care of our neck like how we take care of our face.

Steps for Neck care

1. Use facial cleanser to wash the neck

2. I) After the cleanser, man needs to massage with shave cream then shave daily

2. Ii)After the cleanser, women need to Scrub twice a week on neck.

3. Three times a week facial masks

3. toner/misting Gel

4. Gel Serum

5. Moisturizing Gel

Massage Your Neck

1.http://www.youtube.com/watch?v=DtWGPPY0LJ0&feature=related

2.http://www.youtube.com/watch?v=NWTJI03xPl0

Hope you all have relax with the above neck massage.

See you in next recipe.

12. Eye Care or OIC

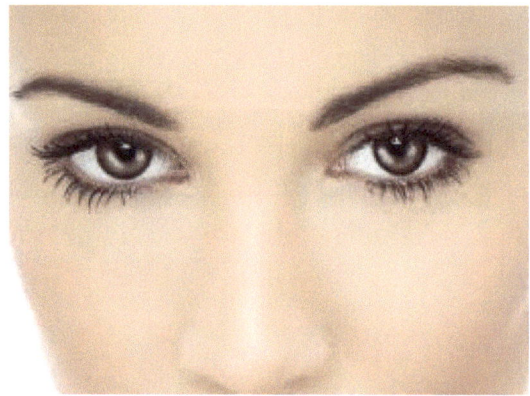

Fruits & Food for eye

1. Carrots
2. Wolfberries
3. Bell peppers
4. Apples
5. Broccoli
6. Brussels sprouts

Eye Care for people who use computer

1. After 20 to 30 minutes, look at green plant at distance away, blink serveral times
2. Blink 12 to 15 times every minutes
3. Exercise your eyes by close your eye and roll them clockwise & anticlockwise with inhale & exhale then open your eyes slowly
4. Rub your palm become warm & cover eyes with the warm palm for a minutes to relax your eyes
5. Splashing water on face to refresh your face during breaks
6. A few minutes of walks during breaks to relax

Watch this to relax your eyes

1.http://www.youtube.com/watch?v=31wFweYz910&feature=related

Share funny jokes with you

1.http://www.youtube.com/watch?v=dMH0bHeiRNg

See you in next recipe!

13. Facial Advice

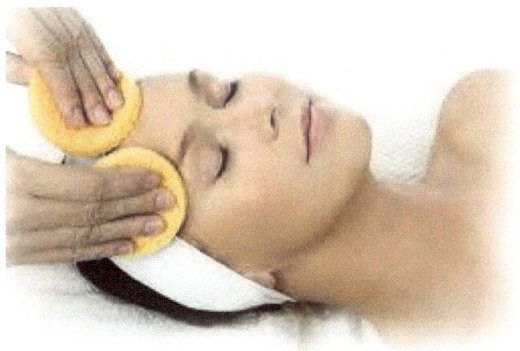

How are you doing my friends?

Today i am sharing with you why men & women need to do facial even we wash our face daily?

Why sometime we use the facial product it hasn't give the results we wants?

Personally, at least i do facial once a month. If those who have pigmentation they need to do facial at least 3 weeks once and for acne skin they need to go for treatments twice a month.

Why we need to go facial?

Actually, in the modern environment, it is full of dust that is why it blocks our face. Therefore, if we do not go for facial no matter what product we use our face will not absorb.

You may try after facial then you continuous use good product which recommended by beautician then you will see younger & fresher look faster.

Well, you need to choose good beautician who really help you to treat your face with good products & not just about earning your money.

They will give lots of useful inside out advice to you to keep you young & healthy.

Furthermore, those good beauticians will help you to massage your face probably in order to avoid wrinkles.

Hope you have shinning & happy & confidence face which will bring tons of luck & prosperity to you!

See you in next recipe!

14.FEET CARE

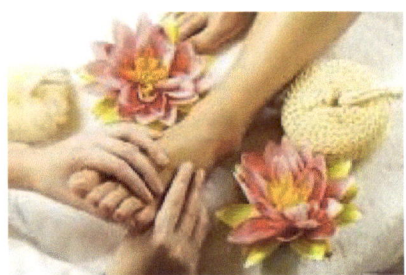

My dear friends, is your feet happy?

Hahaha.. are you looking at your feet now..

Smell good? Wow.. i expect many funny answer from all of you.

I used to call my feet "HONG KONG" feet and i don't know why normally people use to joke with feet by saying "HONG KONG" feet.

Do you have any answer?

We normally overlook our feet.

Actually we need to take good care of our feet too.

Here are some of the things that I am doing in order to repair my "HONG KONG" feet.

I clean my feet properly when i bath, then i will apply lotion to my feet.

I know you are laughing on lotion also on my feet.

Basically, I use lotion for my full body from inside to outside.

As you can see my results, therefore i am very confident on this lotion.

Besides, every morning i will have full body exercise for 20 minutes, it includes my feet too.

See you in next recipe!

http://www.youtube.com/watch?v=ZPlvpN-7xyI&feature=re

15.Arm care

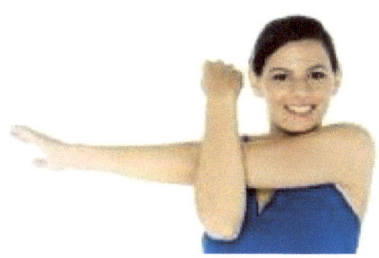

Hello to my friends here.

Today, i am going to share with you on the arm care.

Actually, my arm care is simple.

I just do the same steps as what i did for my face.

Normally, people will overlook on the arm care. However, if you observe & take care on your own arm, you will notice that your skin under or above the arm will be improved.

Hope this remind you on your arm care.

See you in next recipe.

16. TYRE STORY

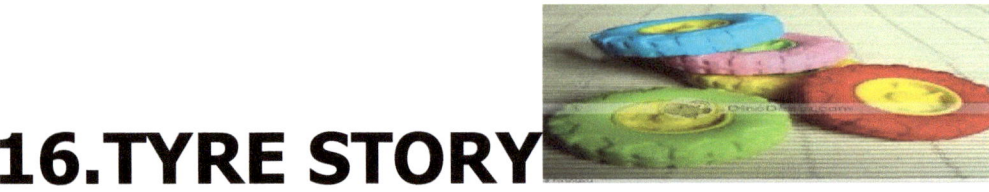

Today, I am going to share with you a true tyre story of mind.

My friend & I have a conversation as below:

My friend: Your shape is round with tyre..(Immediately, my mind imagine myself round like tyre)

Me: Ooooops is it?

(In my mind, I said Oh shit many layers of tyre, how do I get rid of it?)Hahaha

My friend: You need to do something about it. I am your friend that is why I wanted to tell you this.

Me: Thank you

My dear friends, after I had the above conversation I plan to go home after work to do something about it.

As I went home, I know my friend she told me that with good intention. She really wanted to help me as I undergoing some complicated personal matters about 2 years ago.

Since then I have created my own set of personal technique for ME by divided myself into many departments. You are wondering what department I meant right?

1. Mind
2. Eat
3. Exercise
4. Body
5. Face
6. Hand
7. Leg
8. Arm
9. Shape
10. Skills
11. Knowledge
12. Investment
13. Venture future business
14. Sharing
15. Reading

All the above are running concurrently & continuously.

17.Clapping hand

If you are happy and you know it Clap your hand X2 ....very familiar song..and NOW you clap your hand 5 times before you continue reading

Yes, we used to sing this song when we were small girls or boys.

Do you know that Clapping hand is an exercise and it creates good health & circulate our blood on our hand too?

Normally, after i wake up i drink a glass of water then clap my hand and start with my 20 minutes exercise.

If you are curious what sort of 20 minutes exercise then stay tune with me while i prepare my personal video on those very effective & healthy exercise..

Yesterday, I went for investment training. The trainer has mentioned that by clapping our hand it will extend our life for 2 years. Well, i definitely agree with him.

Guess what happened?

All the participants clap their hand as loud as possible. In our daily life, this is an encouragement to others & creates health to ourselves too.

Actually, i have practiced by clapping my hand in the morning ever since i have read one article from newspaper which mentioning that this is a secret of a man who lives until 100 years.

Hope you guys enjoy these articles & see you in next recipe!

18. Rainbow soup

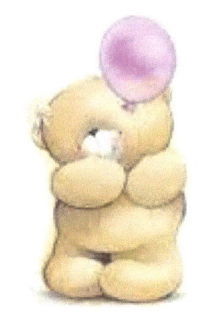

Thank You!

A Forever Friends Giftbook

My dear friends,

Do you like to drink soup?

I like rainbow vegetable soup because it is with all different type of colours.

It is naturally with high fiber & high antioxidants.

Actually, my results are combination of everything...

Now you see how much effort i have put in to get the younger results..

Hope you enjoy my secret recipe. Wish you have good health as the young looking come together with good health...

See you in next recipe :D

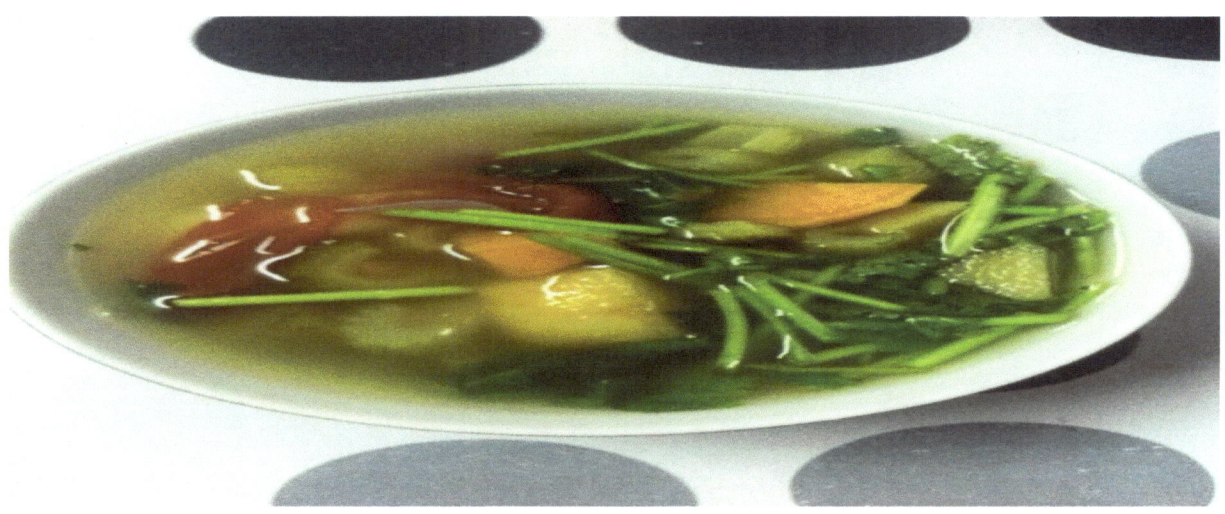

19.Beauty Bath

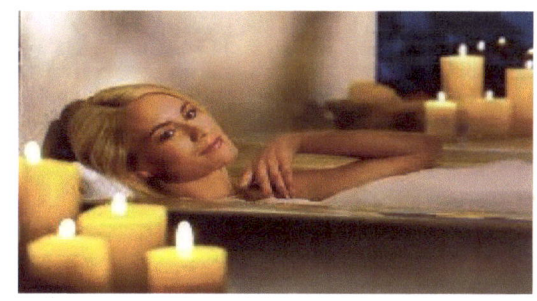

Really excited to see you here!

How many times you take bath a day?

The following are some guidance on how we take bath..

It is funny right?

Yeah it is funny, enjoyable, relaxing during bath..

I love take bath..

a) Temperature-I normally take cold bath, if there is a need i take the temperature from 35'C to 37'C.

To protect the soft & supple skin the above is the best temperature for bath.

2.How long? Avoid too long, about 1/2 to one hour to have good health.

3.Frequency-One or twice a day of bath.

4.Sequence-1st,wash the face,2nd, wash the body,3rd, wash hair.

You may ask why, wash the face first, as we walk into the bathroom, if we turn on the temperature of the water, the temperature will cause our skin open to dirt.

5.Type of skin-Dry skin use the shower cream, oily skin & normal skin use the shower gel which is fresh.

6.Protection after bath-Immediately, after the bath put on lotion to stop the lost of water from skin which could maintain the soft & supple skin.

7.Avoid-Avoid take bath after meal, so that the digestion of food can be done properly & the stomach is still firm.

Well, my dear friends hope you enjoy, relax on bath.

See you in next recipe.

20.Sun block

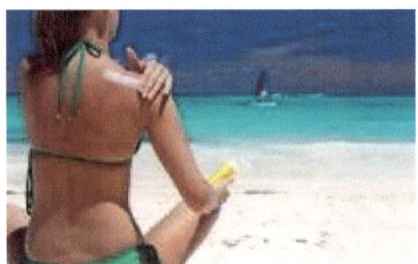

Hey you are wondering like AUSTIN POWER on what i am sharing today...

Guess with the below picture..

Yes, you are right! It is SUN BLOCK.

Are you using sun block, probably you will say yes or you will say i use it only if i go to seaside under the hot sun right.

Actually, every day after i use the facial product i put on sun block

With UV protection & SPF30 or higher.

As you know, if we are standing under the hot sun without sun block our skin will get burn & peeling off.

Therefore, we wear Sun Block under hot sun to avoid burning UVB rays which will cause aging or skin cancer.

That is why, i will get melt like an ice under the hot sun so i have to use umbrella if i am under hot sun.Hahaha..

Tell you one story, my friend she went for holiday and she brought along the SUN BLOCK and she applied the sun block so that she could go to seaside & sit there comfortably.

After a few hour under the hot sun at the seaside she went to toilet.

Suddently, she realised that her face in black & skin peeling off...

She was wondering why?

You guess what happen?

Then,she checked the expired date of the sun block; she found that the sun block was expired.

Hope you protect your skin with the sun block.

See you tomorrow..

21.Funny Slim

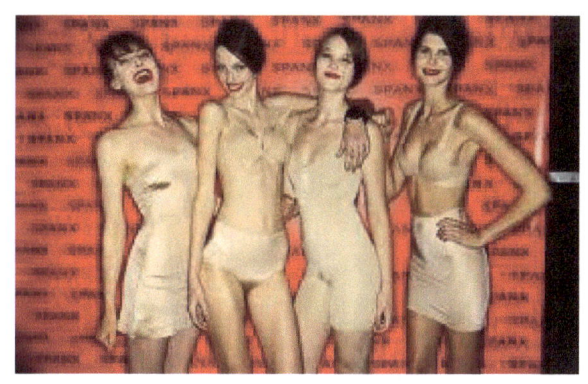

Very excided because i share some perfect shape girls photos,right?

Do you know why i share these?

Actually, anyone could get the same shape as these girls.

I used to be round round like a ball...

You wonder how could i slim down with the shape i want..

Every morning i will wear the above undergarments and do the exercise..eventually after a few weeks i got the shape that i want..

Do you want that? You can have it too..

Therefore, i do not need to wear the undergarments from day to night..I just wear it for exercise only..

Well don't get me wrong i still wear my internal beauty ok...

Cheers & looking forward to see you in next recipe..

You may visit to exercise with the following music so that you enjoy doing exercise with music..

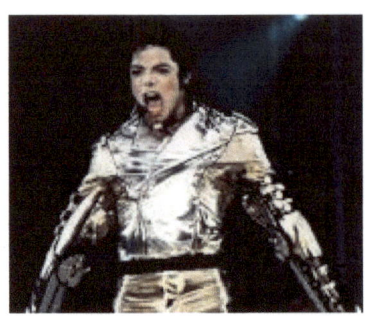

22.MJ drinks

Who is this?

I am sure you know who is he.

Today my sharing is about MJ.

Whooops what is the linkage between MJ versus natural young recipe???

Do you know what is MJ drinks..

Hahaha... MJ drinks very interesting yes or yes?

MJ drink is the mixture of Grass jelly(Cincao) and Soya.

Therefore is a black & white drinks.Wow ...One world one dream!!

It tastes good & good for creating youthful skin & natural health benefits because Cincao & soya with high antixoxidant!

My dear friends on top of Agel products i do drinks MJ drinks quite often.

See you in next recipe!

Tar Tar!!

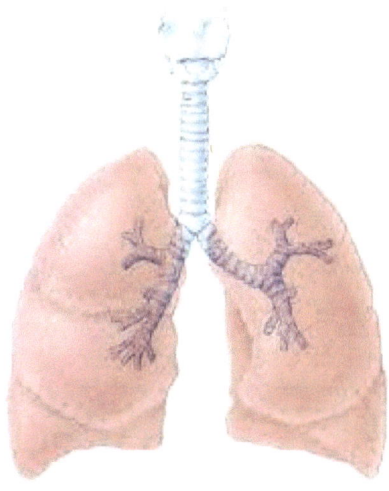

23.Food for lungs

a) **cauliflower, broccoli, and watercress**
It helps to stop the progression of lung cancer in both human and animal studies.

b) **Pomegranate Juice3.Apples**
Pomegranate juice and extract slow the growth of lung tumors. Pomegranates contain many antioxidants including ellagic acid, which is gaining strides in cancer research.

c) **Onions**
Onions provide vitamin C, vitamin B6, and other critical nutrients. These essential nutrients give the body all the power it needs to heal itself. They also have anti-cancer properties also. Another component in onions is quercetin, a natural anti-oxidant. That antioxidant has research behind it showing it helps prevent lung diseases including cancer.

d) **White Grapefruit**
Naringin, a flavonoid in grapefruit, inhibits the activation of a cancer causing enzyme. White grapefruit contains a high amount of this flavonoid, though pink grapefruit has some along with the antioxidant lycopene. Grapefruit is especially good at cleansing the lungs after quitting smoking.

e) **Turmeric**
This spice is related to ginger with many of the same benefits. It also contains curcumin, a compound that encourages the self-destruction of cancer cells

f) **Pumpkin** – Another food rich in vitamin A from beta carotene and vitamin C, like carrots.

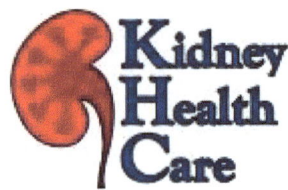

24. Kidney Care

Have you wonder what are the food good for kidney care?

Me too i am wondering which type foods good for kidney.

You may try the following:

a) Red bell peppers

Red bell peppers are a good choice for those concerned about kidney health, because they're low in potassium. In addition, they add color and taste to any dish, while packing a generous portion of vitamins A, C, B6, folic acid and fiber. They also contain the antioxidant lycopene, which protects against certain types of cancer.

b) Cabbage

Inexpensive cabbage is a great addition to your eating plan, because it's also high in vitamins K and C, high in fiber and a good source of vitamin B6 and folic acid, yet it's low in potassium, so it's especially kidney-friendly.

c) Cauliflower

Another kidney-friendly super food is cauliflower. This cruciferous vegetable brings lots of vitamin C to your plate, along with folate and fiber. In addition it contains compounds that help your liver neutralize toxic substances.

d) Garlic

Garlic is good for reducing inflammation and lowering cholesterol. It also has antioxidant and anti-clotting properties. (Cooking garlic will not affect its antioxidant properties, but it will reduce its anti-clotting and anti-inflammatory effects.)

e) Onion

Another popular food used for seasoning is the onion. Onion is full of flavonoids, particularly quercetin. Flavonoids are natural chemicals that prevent the deposit of fatty material in blood vessels and add pigmentation (color) to plants. Quercetin is a powerful antioxidant that is believed to help reduce heart disease and protect against many forms of cancer. It also has anti-inflammatory properties.

f) Apples

An apple a day really does help keep the doctor away! High in fiber and anti-inflammatory properties, apples help reduce cholesterol, prevent constipation, protect against heart disease and decrease your risk of cancer.

g) Cranberries

Cranberries are great for preventing urinary tract infections, because they make urine more acidic and help keep bacteria from attaching to the inside of the bladder. They've also been shown to protect against cancer and heart disease.

h) Blueberries

These tasty berries get their blue color from antioxidant compounds called anthocyanidins. Blueberries get high marks for nutrition, thanks to natural compounds that reduce inflammation and lots of vitamin C and fiber. They also contain manganese, which contributes to healthy bones.

i) Raspberries

Raspberries contain a compound called ellagic acid, which helps neutralize free radicals. The berry's red color comes from antioxidants called anthocyanins. Raspberries are packed with fiber, vitamin C and manganese. They also have plenty of folate, a B vitamin. Raspberries have properties that help stop cancer cell growth and the formation of tumors.

j) Strawberries

Strawberries are rich in two types of antioxidants, plus they contain lots of vitamin C, manganese and fiber. They have anti-inflammatory and anti-cancer properties and also help keep your heart healthy.

k) Cherries

Cherries are filled with antioxidants and phytochemicals that protect your heart. When eaten daily, they have been shown to reduce inflammation.

l) Red grapes

The color in red grapes comes from several flavonoids. These are good for your heart, because they prevent oxidation and reduce the chance of blood clots. One flavonoid in grapes, resveratrol, may boost production of nitric oxide, which increases muscle relaxation in blood vessels for better blood flow. Flavonoids also help protect you from cancer and prevent inflammation.

m) Egg whites

Did you know that egg whites are pure protein? They provide the highest quality protein there is, along with all of the essential amino acids. If you're on the kidney diet, it's good to note that egg whites have less phosphorus than other protein sources, such as egg yolks or meats.

n) Fish

Another high-quality source of protein is fish. Both the American Diabetes Association and the American Heart Association recommend that you include fish in your meal plan two or three times a week. Besides being a great source of protein, fish contains anti-inflammatory fats called omega-3s. These healthy fats help prevent diseases, such as cancer and heart disease. They also help lower LDL (the bad cholesterol) and raise HDL (the good cholesterol).

The types of fish that have the most omega-3s are salmon, albacore tuna, mackerel, herring and rainbow trout.

o) Olive oil

Research has shown that people in countries where olive oil is used instead of other types of oils tend to have lower rates of cancer and heart disease. This is believed to be due to olive oil's many good components: oleic acid, an anti-inflammatory fatty acid which protects against oxidation and polyphenols and antioxidant compounds that prevent inflammation and oxidation.

Use virgin or extra virgin olive oil – they're higher in antioxidants. Olive oil can be used in cooking or to make salad dressing, as a dip for bread and as a marinade for vegetables.

http://www.facebook.com/YoungRecipe?ref=hl#!/YoungRecipe/app_138996027389

25.Laugh to young

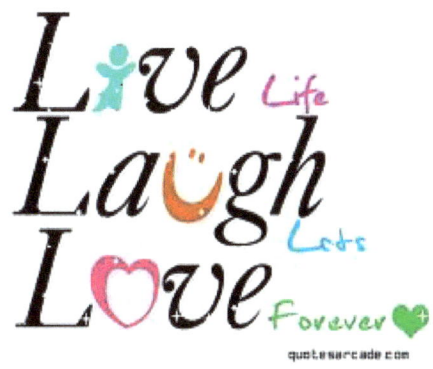

Yes, laughter..

How often you laugh?

Have laugh until like the picture below or the cheek & stomach is fully exercise together?Watch this http://www.youtube.com/watch?v=81NeQJWGYJY

Laughter bring us:

1. health
2. joy
3. release stress
4. lower blood preassure
5. increase blood flow
6. exercise abdominal,respiratory,facial,leg & back muscles

My dear friends, lets enjoy the laughter together!!

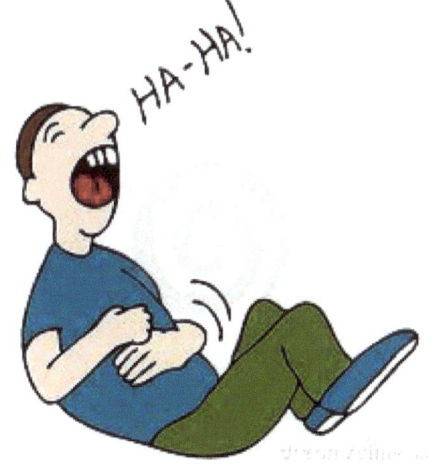

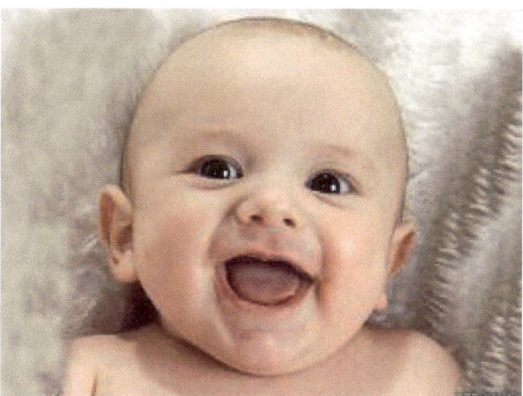

26. MAINTAIN HEALTHY HAIR CARE

Do you know actually it is all about what we eat which contribute to the healthy hair.

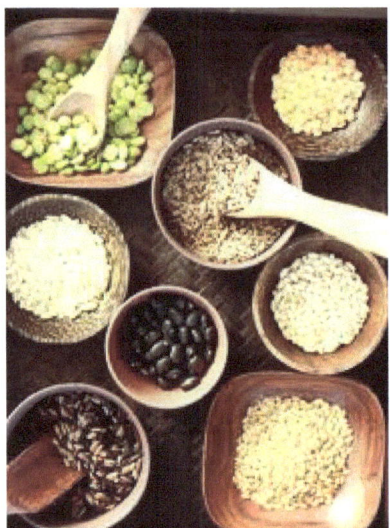Formula to have healthy hair = 5 whole grains(whole wheat bread etc) + protein(tofu/soya etc) + (bean/fish)IRON+ Walnuts/almonds + tomatoes

See you in next recipe.

27.Merry Go Round?

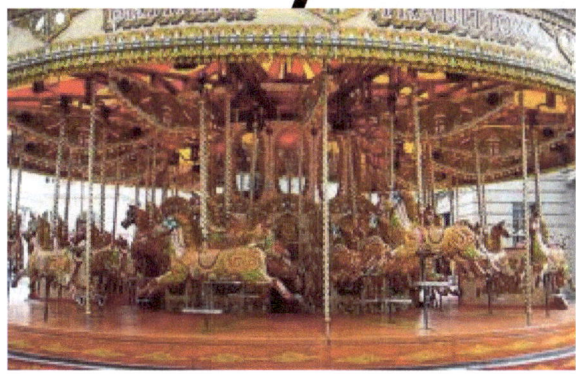

Hello everyone, wish you start with Merry go round day ahead!!

You doubted why the merry go round picture is here right?

Let me share with you how i take my breakfast,lunch, dinner...

Normally, i eat little each time i avoid give burden to my body machine, because i understood if i overloaded my body machine then eventually it needs to send for repair..

I still remembered when i was young my grandmother told me..you have to finish all the food on the plate or else your face will be urgly with pimple...Hahaha.. i think you guys heard the similar comments before correct.

In actual fact, we need to maintain our body machine by taking care carefully, avoid overload the stomach because the machine need to work harder.

Imagine the machine work harder means the machine life will be shorter.

That is why my colleagues saw me eat 1st round,2nd round & 3rd round & each round is little bit...

My 1st round is fruits,2nd round is food,3rd round is drinks..

See you in next Recipe..

28. BMI

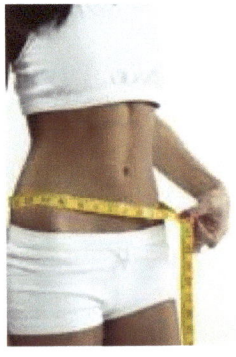

Morning :)

Such a lovely Sunday morning.

Today topic is BIG MONEY IPHONE(BMI)??What???

It is BODY mass index (BMI).

What is your BMI?

Normally, if i pass by a weighting machine in shopping mall, guess what i will do?

Hahaha.. first i look around like james bond..

Then i start take off my shoes, remove some heavy stuff which is in my pockets.

Don't misunderstand.. i will not take off my clothes ok...

So i will measure my weight & check my BMI..

I do monitor my BMI because i want to maintain my ideal BMI in order to stay away from diseases.

My dear friends, find out your BMI before it is too late and FIT & GRN can help us to achieve the ideal BMI too..

http://www.naturalyoungrecipe.com/?page_id=29

The below is the BMI calculator link.

You may check your BMI immediately.

http://www.nestle.com.my/Nutrition_Health_Wellness/wellness_quiz_and_tools/Pages/bmi_calculator.aspx

29.MILK BABY

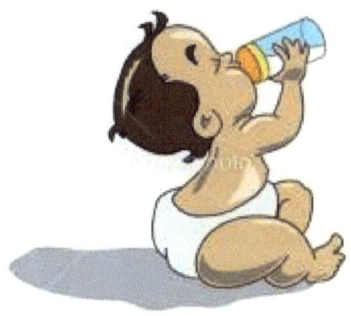

Hello! Cute big big baby...

You wonder why i put a baby picture here right?

Guess what is today topic...

Baby??

Ok ok...today topic is MILK.

How many of you are still drinking milk?

I am still drinking milk like baby..Whooops.. not my mum's milk ok....don't get me wrong ya..

Hahaha.. i still drink a glass of milk a day..

Everthing we eat or drink is reasonable portion only...

Why i drink milk?

Benefits of milk:

    1.Skin
    2.Bone health
    3.Teeth etc

I am sure you would be able read why milk is good for skin,bone,teeth...

Well i hope you enjoy a glass of milk a day...

See you in next recipe..

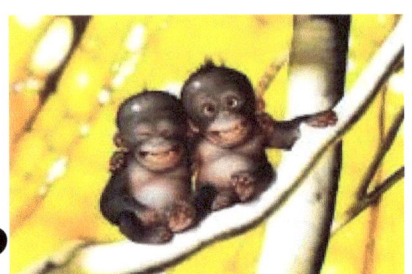

30. SMILE?

Have you come across someone ask you why you **SMILE**, it is weird?

Probably, I give my SMILE so often. Hee hee hee..

Guess what my answer is.

Why you are not SMILLING? it is weird.

Then, we have BIG LAUGH together!!

How often you exercise your face?

What exercise face???

You are wondering what I am talking about, correct?

Yeah.. Exercise your face.

Do you know exercise your face is a **Secret** of have young looking too.

Our facial muscles is attached to bone & muscles with skin.

As you smile it tones and lifts the face & taking the skin with it.

With face exercise you are pushing & pulling on a skin with benefits way & increase the blood circulation which permit more oxygen & nutrients to reach the cells of skin.

IT is **10 times** more **oxygen** goes to a contracting skin muscle than normal.

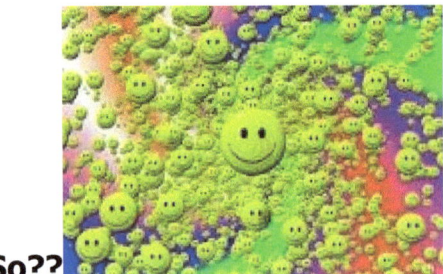

So??

SMILE is a gift to others & yourself too.

31.Funny Oats

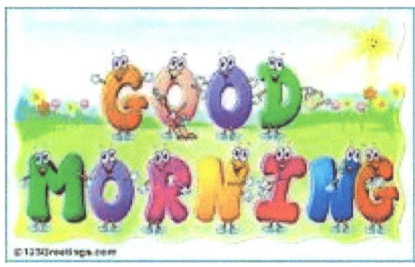

My dear friends. Have you had your breakfast..

What you have today?

Do you have different type of breakfast everyday...

I have different types of breakfast like all of you too like noodles,bread,nasi lemak,cereal,tosey etc

The choice of my breakfast is depend on what i had previous dinner..

Do you clean your car engine if your car engine is full of dirt; can the engine function if the engine is full of dirt?

Hahaha car engine again?? :)

Will you reduce your car engine burden so that your car engine can function well?

If i had very oily & fried food previous day i will eat oats to detox & i will clean my body machine with oats in the next morning.

Everyone know eat oats help you to lower your blood cholesterol, because of high fibre content it protecting us from bowel cancer.

If you have high cholesterol level take the oats daily besides the doctors advices.

Hahaha..let me share my laughter to you. Why?

Because i have created this oats recipe to help myself so that i like oats..

AND i used to keep it secretly.. because my friends said i am weird..

NOW i saw result so I hope it helps you too..

YOU MAY HAVE GOOD LAUGH FIRST!! :D

Oats Recipes

1. Mix oats with cereal
2. Mix oats with drinks like Milo,hot chocholate,coffee,horlic
3. Mix oats with celery,wolfberry,ginger,carrot,milk
4. Mix oats with raisin,almond

Wish you have EXECELLANT natural young & health everyday.

32.Big Big CUP

Hahaha are you curious what i am sharing today?

Lets make a guess!

Ok ok to avoid your neck became like "giraffe neck" ; today topic is drinking water.

Guess how much water i drinks a day?

I knew you will give the right answer, 6 to 8 glass of water.

How many of you have done that?

Hahaha i knew you may forgot or too busy or dislike drinking water..

Steps of drinking water:

1. You may drink the 6 to 8 glasses of water in 4 or 5 times with a bigger mug. (That is why my colleagues use to laugh at my BIG BIG CUP) :)

2. Avoid drink water before you sleep or else you will have puffy eyes then you need cucumber or eye masks to help you to clear that

3. You may drink water with fruit juice.

4. By drinking the jus it helps you to clear your patches on the face & antiaging & maintain your internal organ as young as your face.

5. follow whatever steps you are doing as normal

33.Funny Exercise

Hey good morning...

How do you feel today?

Feeling happy,relax,comfortable...

I am sure you are looking forward to see what is the next secret in this recipe , correct ?

Actually, Exercise is simple.

You are wondering what is combination exercise?

Lets brain storm how many types of exercise is involving the whole body movement together.

The purpose of exercise is to get the results of healthy & young forever.

Let me share with you what type of exercise i do.

I make sure my whole body has all the movement together when i do exercise.

I am sure everyone can do these because it is simple. We all know how to run,jump,shake hands & legs,move up & down,move our head.

Just that simple..

Type of exercise:

1.Combination Exercise-Everytime i do the exercise with my leg,hands,body together with the simple combination of above.

2.Run-Everytime i run my hand is moving together & my body move together.

3.Run Stairs-I run up & down the stairs with the the same movement that i did in running.

4.Walking-I walk with full body movement too.

Now i ask you can you do these?

I think we can do that daily with flexible time because we walk everyday from one place to another.

Sometime we climb the stairs to building, i see the stairs as my tool to get healthy & young so i do walk up the stairs purposes instead of taking the lift.

Hope everyone get some simple tips to do exercise daily in order to achieve excellent health stay forever young with

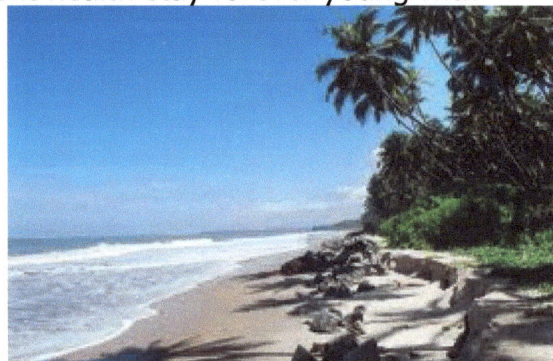

family.

It is time to say bye bye now ..although i wish to share more and i also know time is precious.

Well this bye bye is temporary...I knew you will miss me because i am going to share my next Natural young recipe.

Stay tune :)